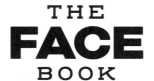

THE
FACE
BOOK

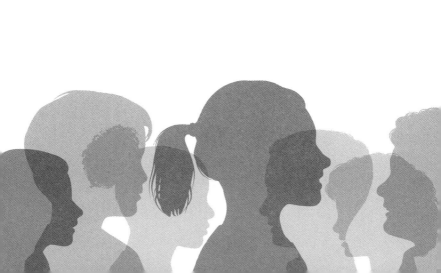

DR. L. DOUGLAS KNIGHT

THE
FACE
BOOK

FUNCTIONAL
AND
COSMETIC
EXCELLENCE
IN ORTHODONTICS

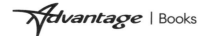

Published by Advantage Books, Charleston, South Carolina.
An imprint of Advantage Media.

ADVANTAGE is a registered trademark, and the Advantage colophon is a trademark of Advantage Media Group, Inc.

Printed in the United States of America.

10 9 8 7 6 5 4 3 2 1

ISBN: 978-1-64225-620-8 (Hardcover)
ISBN: 978-1-64225-619-2 (eBook)

Library of Congress Control Number: 2023909874

Book design by Analisa Smith.

This publication is designed to provide accurate and authoritative information in regard to the subject matter covered. It is sold with the understanding that the publisher is not engaged in rendering legal, accounting, or other professional services. If legal advice or other expert assistance is required, the services of a competent professional person should be sought.

Advantage Books is an imprint of Advantage Media Group. Advantage Media helps busy entrepreneurs, CEOs, and leaders write and publish a book to grow their business and become the authority in their field. Advantage authors comprise an exclusive community of industry professionals, idea-makers, and thought leaders. For more information go to **advantagemedia.com**.

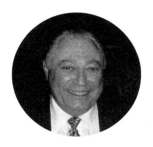

TO DR. RONALD H. ROTH

A guiding light in the realm of orthodontics. Your wisdom, expertise, and unwavering support have shaped me into the clinician I am today. Thank you for sharing your knowledge and instilling in me a passion for excellence. This book stands as a testament to your mentorship, a tribute to the profound impact you've had on my journey.

TO ALL MY OTHER MENTORS

Dr. Jeffrey McClendon – Restorative Dentist, Dr. Rick Roblee – Orthodontist, Dr. Carl Roy – Orthodontist, Dr. Paul Rigali – Orthodontist, Dr. Jeff Okeson – TMJ Dentist, Dr. Larry Jerrold – Orthodontist, Dr.

David Hatcher - Oral and Maxillofacial Radiologist, Dr. Bob Williams - Orthodontist, Dr. Ron Roncone - Orthodontist, Dr. Vince Kokich – Orthodontist, Dr. Ralph Green – Oral Surgeon, Dr. Andy Girardot – Orthodontist, Dr. Domingo Martin – Orthodontist, Dr. Renato Cocconi – Orthodontist, Dr. Mirco Raffaini – Oral Surgeon, Dr. Jorge Ayala – Orthodontist, Dr. Joseph Van Sickels – Oral Surgeon. Your guidance has paved the path before me. Your mentorship, encouragement, and belief in my potential have been instrumental in shaping my career. Your lessons and insights have become the foundation upon which I've built my expertise in orthodontics. This book is dedicated to each one of you, grateful for the invaluable wisdom you've imparted.

TO MY WIFE

Your tireless commitment to managing the office with compassion and precision has transformed our workplace into an environment where patients feel welcomed and cared for. Your impeccable organization and attention to detail ensure that everything runs seamlessly behind the scenes, allowing me to focus on creating beautiful smiles. Thank you for being the backbone of our success.

TO THE PATIENTS CONTEMPLATING ORTHODONTIC TREATMENT

This book is dedicated to you, the individuals embarking on a transformative journey towards a beautiful and healthy smile. Your courage, curiosity, and commitment to improving your oral health is inspiring.

Within these pages, I strive to empower you with knowledge and understanding, as I believe an informed patient is an empowered patient. I acknowledge the questions, concerns, and doubts that may accompany your decision, and it is my purpose to provide clarity, guidance, and reassurance.

I recognize the impact that orthodontic treatment can have on your self-esteem, confidence, and overall well-being. Your willingness to embark on this path reflects your belief in the power of a radiant smile.

May this book serve as a roadmap, enlightening you about the intricacies of orthodontics and the possibilities that lie ahead. With each chapter, I aim to equip you with the knowledge and understanding necessary to make informed decisions about your orthodontic journey.

WISHING YOU A FULFILLING AND REWARDING ORTHODONTIC EXPERIENCE, DOUG.

CONTENTS

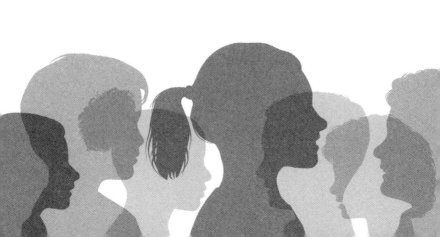

FOREWORD

In this era of direct-to-consumer advertising, patients seeking "straight teeth and a beautiful smile" are inundated with an overwhelming number of treatment options. Many of the options, while good for companies, are not good for patients.

There is much more to orthodontics than simply straightening teeth. When teeth are moved without an individualized treatment plan by a trained specialist, serious dental problems can occur including gum, joint, and bite problems.

The question becomes, how can patients know which treatment plan is in their best interests?

Dr. Knight has provided excellent guidance for the orthodontic consumer to understand how to avoid treatment problems and achieve excellent results. To achieve exceptional results, there is a need for a systematic and objective approach to orthodontic treatment which is outcome directed. Brilliantly simplified and listed by Dr. Knight are the *required* outcomes of exceptional orthodontic treatment.

- Dental aesthetics and facial harmony
- Functional occlusions
- Airway size adequacy
- Patient satisfaction
- TMJ health
- Gum health

With this book patients will have the information they need to choose treatment and doctors to avoid complications and achieve excellent results.

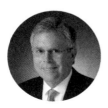

—Dr. Bill Arnett

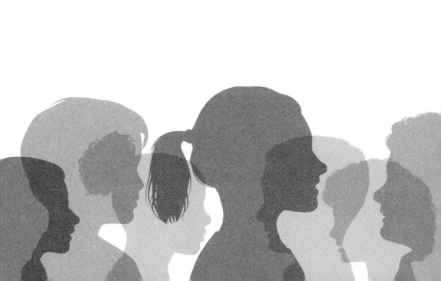

My Origin Story

In 1989, I was a young dentist in the army, not too far out from my year of general practice residency. For the most part, I was pleased with my career choice. Dentistry is complex and interesting and a great way to help people. But I was feeling a little troubled. I fixed people's mouths one tooth at a time, even making ugly teeth pretty again, but I didn't feel completely satisfied. Many patients had more complex problems beyond needing simple fillings or crowns. It was rewarding to restore people's teeth, but I wanted to provide more. It seemed I was getting to the limit of everything I could learn about general dentistry. I wanted to provide a more comprehensive plan of treatment that would provide the correction of a patient's underlying problems, something that benefited a patient far more than just restoring teeth and that would be more rewarding and fulfilling to me on a daily basis.

As luck or providence would have it, that "something new" I was looking for presented itself on a very normal day during a continuing education course at Walter Reed Army Medical Center. Dr. Ron Roth had come to speak. I had heard of him through colleagues and comments by the military mojos of the dental corps. All I really knew was that he was an orthodontist who practiced in California and lectured all over the world.

As his big, booming voice filled the room, he talked about guiding the growth and development of teeth that made aesthetic-looking faces. He discussed bites that supported muscles in a relaxed position and provided comfortable jaw joints and even helped with migraines. He described how to provide treatment that would enhance airways to prevent sleep apnea and improve attention-deficit hyperactivity disorder (ADHD) in children. I knew orthodontics was about straightening teeth, but what Dr. Roth described was much bigger than that. This was about life-changing, life-enhancing effects that stayed with people forever and improved their overall health in countless ways. It gave people a better future. This was the thing I had a hunch about but had never heard anyone explain in detail before. He presented clear and cutting-edge data that supported everything he said. It made so much sense. It was a comprehensive, interdisciplinary, goal-oriented approach to the treatment of the entire system. This approach sought to increase the longevity of the dentition, periodontium, and the joints and promote healthy function of the muscles. Quantifiable goals for dental and facial aesthetics were outlined. I had never been taught so much in one lecture. I had one of those movie-scene moments where I knew exactly what I wanted to do. My life changed that day, and I decided right then and there that I was going to become an orthodontist. But not just any kind of orthodontist. I was going to follow in Dr. Roth's footsteps and become an orthodontist that helped people in real ways, beyond just straight teeth.

I knew my next step was getting into an orthodontic residency program, but first I had to fulfill my army duties from the Reserve Officer Training Corps scholarship I had received while attending the University of Kentucky. That took a few more years.

All the while, I was building a relationship with Dr. Roth. We had kept in touch, and he was mentoring me. I sought his counsel regularly and eventually was accepted to the New York University Orthodontic Training Program in Manhattan in July 1993. I also did something very unusual for orthodontic residents. I began a two-year postgraduate training program with Dr. Roth while still in my NYU program. It was hard and a little risky. I had to take out loans not only for my NYU tuition but also for our basic living expenses, and now for Dr. Roth's comprehensive course. In addition, I paid for flights to travel back and forth to California, where

Dr. Roth's practice and training center was, multiple times a year.

As hard as it was, I knew I was doing the right thing. I had finally found my path. I strongly desired to know and understand orthodontics at a deeper level. I wanted to be more than a tooth straightener; I wanted to be a real healthcare provider. Dr. Roth noticed. He mentored me every step of the way. Many evenings during my visits to California, he took me out to dinner for an evening of stories and further education. We were just two men, a current and future orthodontist, talking about life and treatment philosophy.

I continued to train with Dr. Roth, and he regularly invited me to attend his Functional Occlusion courses in San Francisco in San Francisco to present real-life cases from my own practice. Pretty soon we began lecturing together, and I became a teacher too. We traveled the world lecturing to other orthodontists about this comprehensive kind of care and maintained a close friendship until his untimely death from cancer in 2005. I was devastated that my mentor and friend had passed too soon, and I became all the more dedicated to our mission as he metaphorically passed the torch to me.

Today, I still run that practice in Radcliff and have a second office in Louisville. I still travel the world teaching other orthodontists and have developed a reputation for seeing some of the most difficult cases in my community. All of this is because of Dr. Roth and the mission we began together decades ago.

How Is FACE Different?

The purpose of this book is to further that mission and educate you, my patients, and the public about the FACE philosophy. In this era of do-it-yourself orthodontics and less expensive, mail-away retainers that don't require you to even set foot in an orthodontist's office, we're getting further and further away from understanding what creates the best long-term outcomes and that straight teeth are only a small part of what makes a healthy, functioning mouth. The general population, and even some dental and orthodontic practices, care mostly about the cosmetic aspect and little about the functional.

My patient population is 60 percent children. Parents want their kids to have the advantages that come with a nice smile, but they also want them to have well-functioning mouths. They don't want them to have problems later in life. But in many cases, they don't know where to turn for help—they don't understand that orthodontics is more than just straight teeth. Straight teeth do not necessarily indicate a healthy and well-functioning bite. They also are not the only metric for an aesthetically pleasing face. We'll get into more details about the goals of FACE orthodontics in the following chapters, but briefly, they are as follows:

- Straight teeth to create a nice smile

- Correcting the bite by treating the way in which the teeth fit together, with the jaw joints in the socket, protects our masticatory system from excessive shifting, trauma, and wear.

- Creating a balanced, proportional, and symmetrical face

- Ensuring the airway has no obstructions or encroachments that might contribute to sleep-disordered breathing

Do-it-yourself orthodontics can't address all the underlying issues that impact a smile, let alone your overall health. It can't correct underlying skeletal discrepancies. It's important to fix those underlying problems to prevent lifelong issues. In some cases, people have their teeth straightened more than once and the underlying problem is never fixed. That's what we're trying to avoid. I want to provide patients with a beautiful smile that creates confidence and delight in how they look and treat any foundational problems that create issues many patients might not even know they have or will develop down the road.

Did you know improper airway or jaw function can cause sleep apnea, migraines, temporomandibular joint disorders (TMJ), and even ADHD? Did you know there are quantifiable metrics we can use to adjust your jaw and lips to create a more pleasing look? Did you know your previously straight teeth might be shifting because your tongue is blocking your airway and you actually have a breathing problem and not just a tooth problem?

It's time we had a more comprehensive view of orthodontics and value the proper functioning of everything else above our shoulders as much as we do our straight teeth. With FACE orthodontic treatment, you won't just get straight teeth. You'll get the assurance that this part of your overall health is operating to

> **It's time we … value the proper functioning of everything else above our shoulders as much as we do our straight teeth.**

its fullest potential so you can too, for the entirety of your life. Thank you for picking up this book and caring to learn more about this vital aspect of your or your child's health. Let's dive into the foundational aspects of the FACE philosophy.

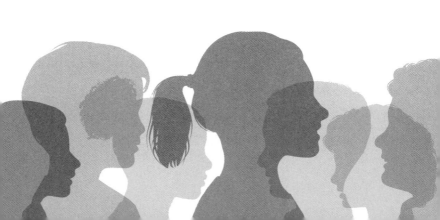

CHAPTER 1

Goal-Oriented Treatment

The Problem

I'm sure you are not surprised to hear that most people go to the orthodontist because they want to straighten their teeth or are looking for some kind of aesthetic service. I understand that we want to look nice. We're only human, right? But just straightening the teeth without addressing underlying issues may cause you many more complex and serious problems in the long run. I bet your TMJ isn't nearly as troubling to you as being embarrassed to smile big and show your teeth if you're unhappy with them. A huge culprit in people's insecurities is their imperfect teeth. So they, or their children, land in my office. One of the things I find myself doing all day long (and a big reason why I decided to write a book) is explaining to people *why* they have crooked teeth or a visibly imperfect bite that gives them anxiety. These things can be a symptom of something bigger, more foundational, but they're often the thing that eventually prompts them to seek care. And of course, children and adolescents come around the time their adult teeth are in and it's time to straighten things out.

I'd estimate that 90–95 percent of the patients I see have no clue about everything that is wrong, whether it's causing problems now or will slowly wear things down over the next twenty years. One of the greatest anecdotal testaments to the FACE philosophy is that the majority of dentists in my area bring their children to my practice. They trust what we're doing here so strongly that they have confidence we'll correct any issues early in their kids' developmental years and set them up with beautiful smiles and functional mouths for life. Even if they don't know how to diagnose it or correct it themselves, they understand this functional piece is essential in the long run.

Part of what sets the FACE treatment philosophy apart is its unique goal-oriented approach. All orthodontics is goal-oriented to some degree, but in most cases, its singular goal is to straighten teeth. Direct-to-consumer companies offer simple, cheap solutions to straighten the teeth, but nothing else. They bombard the airwaves with advertisements that put a lot of pressure on orthodontists to make straightening teeth their main focus and to do it quickly. This couldn't be further from the way FACE orthodontics works. The best description of the FACE philosophy that has been refined over many years by different professionals is this: a comprehensive, interdisciplinary approach to the treatment of the entire system with emphasis placed on the face.

It's comprehensive because it takes into account the whole body and sees your orthodontic health as a piece of that whole. It's interdisciplinary because in the course of FACE orthodontic care, there is a good chance the orthodontist may not be able to fix everything and will need the assistance of a periodontist, restorative dentist, oral surgeon, or an ear, nose, and throat specialist (ENT). I cannot remove a child's enlarged adenoids, but I may diagnose them when I'm evaluating their airway for constrictions. Emphasis is placed on the face because often nothing else matters much to the patient if they don't like how they look and have a functional mouth.

To better understand the different kinds of goals and their importance, there are some other foundational ideas I need to explain first.

The Three Levels of Orthodontic Care

Unlike that succinct description above, three levels of care are not something you'll find on a website or in textbooks. This is something I came up with as I explain and work to simplify these concepts to laypeople every day. Here is all of orthodontics boiled down into three levels of care:

Level one: straighten teeth. The first level of care is the simplest. This is something the DIY aligner companies can do for you, hopefully (though many people eventually end up in my office anyway because they failed in some way and need further treatment, and good luck trying to get the DIY aligner companies on the phone). If you come in with crooked teeth, they're only going to just straighten them for you. If your upper and lower jaw happens to be in good alignment, you might get lucky and the teeth will fit together. But that's only a small percentage of people. Most have a bit of an underlying skeletal problem, and if you only straighten the teeth, chances are they will not fit together properly.

Level two: straighten teeth and correct the bite. The second level of care is where we're going to straighten the teeth and also get them to fit together properly. Teeth should fit together like a zipper or a jigsaw puzzle. The teeth should not hit end against end, which causes all sorts of bigger problems. If you need level-two care, you should see an orthodontist. You cannot get this level of care through a DIY company; any traditionally trained orthodontist can handle it.

Level three: straighten teeth, correct bite, correct jaw-joint position, and evaluate airway, tooth form, smile aesthetics, and facial aesthetics. This is what FACE orthodontics will do for you, everything from levels one and two and then some. Of course, we straighten the teeth and correct the bite. But perhaps your jaw joints are out of the socket. That requires correction of your jaw-joint position to make sure you have a good harmony between the teeth and joints. We'll ensure you have good form on the teeth if they have previously worn down, thus ensuring proper function going forward. Perhaps you have airway problems that may or may not even be discernable to you and you have sleep-disturbed breathing. Or maybe you have what we call a "gummy" smile and show an excessive amount of gum above your upper teeth. This level of care will correct those things as well when the bite is corrected. And lastly, we'll improve your smile and facial aesthetics. There are standards and ways we quantify the ideal facial proportions to create a beautiful face, not just a beautiful smile. We can change your profile, move your jaw forward or backward, and even give you the appearance of fuller lips. This is the kind of comprehensive, life-changing care all modern orthodontics should encompass.

> **There are standards and ways we quantify the ideal facial proportions to create a beautiful face, not just a beautiful smile.**

With this understanding of the levels of orthodontic care in mind, let's discuss the four principles of FACE orthodontics.

The Four Principles

The goals of FACE treatment are guided by four lifelong principles that never change. That's the big difference between goals and principles. Principles were the same twenty years ago, and they'll be the same twenty years from now. These are the building blocks, the fundamentals of anything in dentistry or orthodontics.

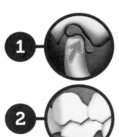

Proper Joint Function
Form of Joints
CO=CR

Functional Occlusion
Form of Occluded Dentition

Anterior Guidance
Form of Teeth
Vertical and Horizontal Overbite

Facial Aesthetics
Ideal Proportions

PRINCIPLE ONE: PROPER JOINT FUNCTION

The jaw joint was made to fit directly into the socket. It's as simple as that. Everything functions better when your jaw is in its socket. A great amount of focus is placed on this aspect of care. An instrument called an articulator is used to evaluate a patient's jaw-joint position. Most orthodontists will check your bite, but it's not properly assessed unless you evaluate it when your jaw joint is actually in the socket.

Splint therapy, also known as occlusal splint therapy or orthotic therapy, is a treatment approach used to manage temporomandibular joint (TMJ) disorders, bruxism (teeth grinding), and other related conditions. The main goal of splint therapy is to provide stability and relief to the temporomandibular joint and its associated structures.

1. Muscle Relaxation: Splints are designed to help relax the muscles around the TMJ. By providing a stable and properly aligned occlusal surface (the way the upper and lower teeth come together), the splint can reduce the strain and tension in the muscles,

allowing them to relax. This relaxation can help guide the condyle into a more favorable position within the socket.

2. Joint Decompression: The use of an occlusal splint can help decompress the TMJ by creating a separation between the upper and lower teeth. This separation reduces the load and pressure on the joint, potentially allowing the condyle to seat more comfortably in the socket.

3. Re-Establishing Normal Function: Splint therapy aims to restore proper occlusal relationships and improve the harmony of the jaw's movements. By doing so, the splint can help realign the condyle within the socket, allowing it to settle into a more optimal position.

It's important to note that the exact effects of splint therapy may vary depending on the individual and the specific condition being treated. The success of splint therapy relies on careful evaluation, diagnosis, and appropriate customization of the splint to meet the patient's needs.

The articulator acts like a jaw-motion simulator to uncover how your teeth truly fit together when the jaw joint is in its proper seated position.

On the next page, you can see a person with severe TMJ. One picture is their "normal" bite, and the second is their bite when it is actually in the socket, which shows how bad it really is. To truly help this person with their TMJ, we need to fix the bite when it's in the socket, its proper position. But as you can see, it's a much bigger job.

Evaluating the bite.

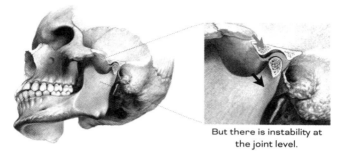

The upper and lower teeth fit each other well in the mouth.

But there is instability at the joint level.

The joint is not in the socket.

Evaluate the bite with the jaw in the socket.

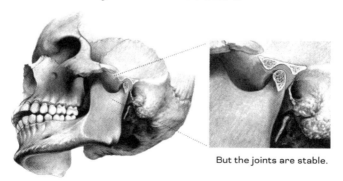

The upper and lower teeth don't fit in the mouth.

But the joints are stable.

The joint is in the socket.

PRINCIPLE TWO: FUNCTIONAL OCCLUSION

Occlusion is the way your teeth meet when your jaws bite together. It is the idea of teeth fitting together like a zipper, as you can see in the graphic below. The tip of one tooth goes down into the little groove of another tooth. That is the way teeth are supposed to fit together to function properly. And like almost everything else I'll mention throughout the book, if this isn't happening, it will create problems. Some may be evident now, and some may not appear for many years.

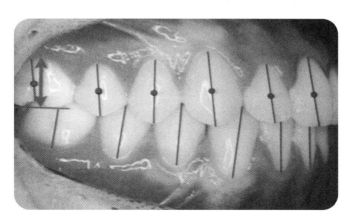

Functional occlusion incorporates the movement of how the jaw moves freely without interference from improper tooth contacts or prematurities upon opening and closing. It is dependent on the jaw joints being in the socket.

PRINCIPLE THREE: ANTERIOR GUIDANCE

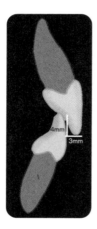

Overbite & Overjet

Overbite 4mm

Overjet 3mm

There is a proper position for your front teeth to be in to function properly when you chew. Both the vertical and horizontal relationship are critical when your jaw opens or moves left and right. This overlap of the front teeth causes the separation of the back teeth when your jaw moves, thus protecting your back teeth from unwanted harmful contacts. When the jaw moves left or right, only your canines should contact, thus preventing any of the back teeth from contacting one another. When your jaw moves straight forward, only the front teeth should contact, once again preventing any of the back teeth from touching. The anterior teeth guide jaw movement and protect the back teeth from harmful interferences. You only want those back teeth to come together when you completely bite down. The front teeth guide everything and prevent all your teeth from wear and tear. If your front teeth do not relate to one another properly, then you have a functional problem. It doesn't matter how perfect and straight they may be. Over time you are at risk of having a problem, such as tooth wear, TMJ, gingival recession, inflammation of the pulp, tooth movement, or a combination of any or all of these.

PRINCIPLE FOUR: FACIAL AESTHETICS

The last principle is about facial balance and the ideal facial proportions. This can differ between societies and races. There may be norms in different cultures that dictate what is perceived as attractive. Some cultures prefer a smaller, set-back lower jaw, while others don't mind a more protrusive one. This also varies between gender. Predictably, men like a more prominent jaw, as that is stereotypically considered masculine in the United States, and women generally don't want a square or more noticeable, strong chin. We'll get into a longer discussion of this in a later chapter, but you can see a graphic on the next page depicting the ideal facial proportions for a Caucasian female. If we drop an imaginary line from the base of the nose, which is perpendicular to the natural forward head posture, we see how the chin is slightly behind this red vertical line. That's where most females in our society generally want to be, with the lower lip right on the line or up to three millimeters ahead of it. The upper lip should rest 2–5 mm in front of this line.

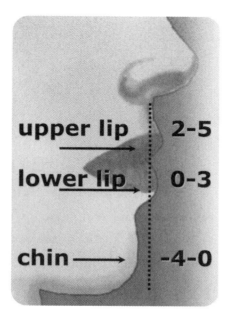

As I said before, these principles are fundamental to dentistry and orthodontics. But whether or not they get addressed is a whole different question. The layperson thinks orthodontics consists of just straightening teeth, which has begun to drive most of the care provided today. People can have ideally straight teeth, but their smile may still not be aesthetically pleasing. Or worse yet, a person with a beautiful smile and straight teeth might be experiencing TMJ pain or sleep-disturbed breathing due to a constricted airway or jaw-joint problem.

Goals

All of this brings us to the goals of FACE treatment. Every patient is different, so the goals of every case are different and potentially infinite. But the four principles remain the same and guide these choices. Having straight teeth is a goal of orthodontics, but if you noticed, it's not actually a principle. Though goals vary greatly, they all revolve around some combination of these factors:

- Dental aesthetics and facial harmony

- Functional occlusion

- Airway

- Long-term stability

- Patient satisfaction

- TMJ health

• Periodontal health

I recently treated a woman who came in and had a big space between her two front teeth, along with other kinds of spacing throughout the mouth. She wanted me to close all the other spacing except the one between her two front, upper teeth, because she really liked that about herself. This is a good example of a goal, closing spacing and straightening teeth, that doesn't violate a principle. It also illuminates a situation that sometimes occurs where the chief concerns of the patient and the orthodontist may differ. It would not have been my choice to keep that front gap, but it was important to her, and patient satisfaction is also a goal. Because FACE orthodontics is an interdisciplinary practice, occasionally patients won't want the recommended procedure or dental work. All of this factors into the personal and unique goals set for each patient, guided by and not violating the four unchanging principles and always aiming to give them level-three orthodontic care that focuses on the entire system.

FACE Treatment

In the course of determining your goals and formulating a plan of treatment, a FACE-trained orthodontist will do two primary things differently. Here is what you can expect:

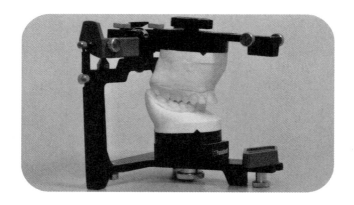

1. Mounted models. Models of your teeth are placed on a jaw-motion simulator (articulator), which I mentioned in principle one, to more accurately and correctly identify how your teeth fit together when the jaw joint is in the socket.

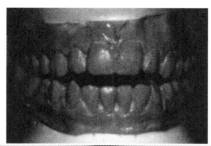

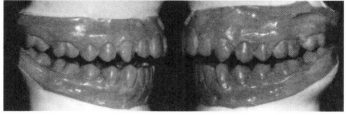

2. Visualized treatment objective (VTO). For every patient, we do computer-generated imaging to go over what their treatment options are. Put simply, we know exactly where the teeth are supposed to be. Using the VTO, we can show them precisely what their options are in order to receive the desired outcome they want. We establish goals in collaboration with the patient so they can visualize what they will look like posttreatment.

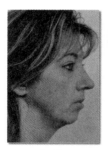
Pre Tx

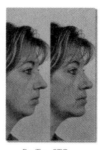
Pre Tx - STO

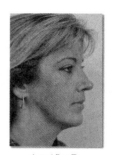
Actual Post Tx

With your goals decided, a treatment plan in place, and the optimism that in the near future you'll look and feel better, you can move forward confidently. In the following chapters, we'll do a deeper dive into the FACE orthodontic treatment philosophy, focusing on achieving optimal facial balance and harmony, in addition to straightening teeth. Through the use of advanced diagnostic tools and treatment techniques, FACE orthodontics strives to provide patients with beautiful smiles that enhance their overall facial appearance and contribute to their long-term oral health and well-being.

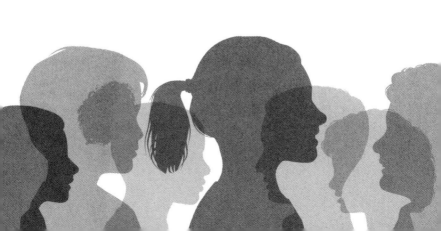

CHAPTER 2

Ideal Facial Aesthetics

What I care about most is helping my patients become the best version of themselves that they can possibly achieve and enjoy improved facial balance and function, along with an outstanding smile and the ability to breathe better, chew better, and live better. I really enjoy seeing how pleased people are with those results. But I wanted to start here with our technical chapters because these lines and measurements that I'll explain below do guide all of our treatment plans when we're deciding where jaws and teeth should be.

Did you know that to some extent, we can quantify beauty? What's reassuring about this approach is that it takes so much of the subjectivity out of planning treatment. It quantifies exactly where the teeth and jaws need to be placed in order to achieve a balanced profile. We know where everything needs to be moved in order to align with societal norms. And the most amazing part is that when you put everything in its proper position for aesthetics, you typically get proper function. Let's get into principle four of FACE orthodontics: facial aesthetics.

Upper Incisors to Anterior Nasal Spine
Up. Inc = ANS

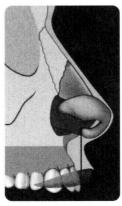

Ideal Upper Lip support

It's important for the teeth to be in the correct position sagittally, front to rear. If somebody's teeth are too far back, they won't support the lip, which of course will affect facial aesthetics. There's an anatomical landmark that we refer to in order to evaluate the proper sagittal position of the upper incisor. It's called the anterior nasal spine. It is a hard tissue structure at the base of the nose and can only be seen radiographically. The upper central incisor should be on or slightly in front of a line dropped vertically from the anterior nasal spine.

We evaluate the vertical position of the teeth as well, and the upper incisors should be about 3–4 mm below a point called upper stomion. Upper stomion is a soft-tissue structure that represents the lowest, most inferior point of the upper lip. If we draw a horizontal yellow line through upper stomion, perpendicular to the teeth, we would like to see the tip edge of the upper incisors 3–4 mm below that line. The tip of the lower incisors should be even with the yellow line because we want a 3–4 mm overlap of the upper incisors to the lower incisors. It's only possible to view these relationships on an X-ray as opposed to seeing them in the mouth.

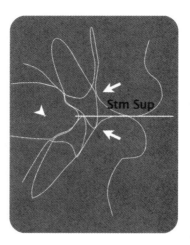

We see all extremes of vertical positioning of teeth. Some people's upper incisors are too high up, and when they smile, you see hardly any of their upper teeth, and with other people, you see the full length of their teeth and a lot of gingival tissue as well.

Let's look at an example. Before treatment, you saw hardly any of this young lady's teeth when she smiled. The teeth were brought down orthodontically to give her more tooth display when she smiles.

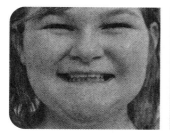 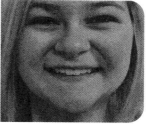

We want to have the proper vertical and hori-zontal overlap of the front teeth so that when the jaw moves forward, the lower teeth contact the back surface of the upper teeth and result in the back teeth separating, thus protecting the back teeth from shear forces and from wearing down. The same scenario occurs when the lower jaw moves left or right. This time, the lower canine contacts the back surface of the upper canine, resulting in the back teeth separating, protecting the back teeth from any harmful contact and wear. This concept of the front teeth contacting during movement in any direction and protecting the back teeth from harmful lateral forces is known as anterior guidance. Wear on any teeth is a sign that something is out of position. If your teeth and jaw joints are in the proper position, tooth wear should not occur.

The position of the lower incisor is set by the upper incisor position, both vertically and horizontally. The most prominent point of the hard tissue of the chin, also known as pogonion, should be in the same vertical plane as the front surface of the lower incisors.

Another relationship that is related to the position of the front surface of the upper incisors is the most inward position of the soft tissue between the lower lip and the chin. This point is called the soft tissue B point. So, the front surface of the upper incisors should be not only in alignment with the anterior nasal spine, but with soft tissue B point as well. It is interesting how all this fits together! These are some guidelines that help us plan treatment. Many patients come in and have multiple problems. As an orthodontist, my brain could go in a million different directions. What should I fix first, and how do I fix it? Having this simple diagram is really beneficial in knowing how to take the most complex cases and create something ideal.

Goals for Treatment

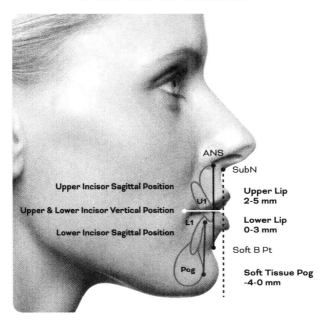

Look at the dotted line in the diagram. That point at the base of the nose is called subnasale. If we were to drop a line perpendicular to this soft-tissue landmark, we would like to see that the upper lip is

2–5 mm ahead of that line. And we want the lower lip on that line or up to 3 mm in front of it. Women generally prefer a softer chin, so I'd want the chin behind that line like the woman in the diagram. And for a stronger chin for men, we want it right at the line or slightly past it. I tell my orthodontic residents when I'm teaching that with these three little lines right here—dotted, black, and white—you can treat most of the cases that you ever come across.

When one part of the system is out of place, it not only affects facial aesthetics but usually function as well. If an upper or lower jaw is retrusive, it will typically impinge upon the airway. This can possibly lead to sleep-disturbed breathing and sleep apnea. I probably see this every day. Our cheeks, lips, and tongue provide forces on our teeth. The tongue provides an outward force, and the cheeks and lips provide an inward force. If there is not enough space for the tongue, we often see the teeth in the front of the mouth pushed forward due to the brain telling the tongue to move forward in order to open the airway, ultimately helping you to breathe. The effects on the teeth are typically spacing and tooth wear on the edges of the front teeth.

We'll get into this deeper in the airway chapter, but I do want to point out how the aesthetic look of the teeth and face are linked to the function of everything else. Patients want to straighten their teeth, but a thorough understanding of the underlying problems aids in making the correct

The aesthetic look of the teeth and face are linked to the function of everything else.

treatment decisions. Often, it's good to ask the question, "How and why are things in the condition they are in?"

In chapter one I mentioned that one thing that sets FACE orthodontists apart is that we do a visualized treatment plan with every patient. We sit down with them to show them in a simulation where the teeth and jaws are supposed to be and what they might expect to look like after treatment. This is where we establish our goals after we've done a full diagnosis and know what the problems are. As I said at the start of the chapter, what we're really doing here is solving systemic problems, but as you can imagine, it's often the visual improvement that gets patients really excited when they see this. I recently saw a six-teen-year-old girl with a very retruded profile. I ran the computer visualization program and showed her and her mom what her profile would look like if we moved her jaw forward (according to our standardized aesthetic proportion diagram above). Until then, she had been withdrawn, a little "too cool" to be at the orthodontist's office. But when she saw what her new profile would look like, a switch went off. She yelled out, "Mom, that's me! That's me with a chin! Look, I have lips. That's what I need. I'm sick and tired of my profile." It's life-changing stuff, especially for these sensitive teenagers.

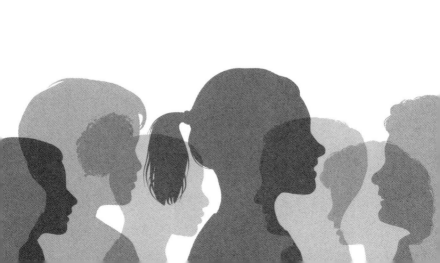

CHAPTER 3

The Form of Teeth

Do you have an aged smile? You likely don't observe this consciously, as you do with wrinkles, but flat, short teeth are a tell-tale sign of aging and make your brain think, "that person is older." Just because you get older does not mean that your teeth should change their shape and form. Your hairline might recede, and you can't do anything about that, but wear on the teeth is preventable. If you have any kind of wear on your teeth, we consider that a dysfunctional occlusion. We want to set up the teeth, jaw, and bite so that everything is functional and there's no wear on the teeth, no bone loss around the teeth, and no gum recession or teeth shifting.

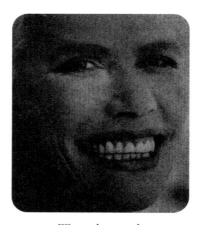

Worn, short teeth.

The form of the teeth is related to the function that they serve. We want to create a relationship between the upper and lower teeth that functions properly without any destructive forces placed on the teeth, jaw joints, or other supporting structures. Proper tooth form increases the longevity, health, and aesthetics of a beautiful smile.

1. Incisors: These are the sharp, chisel-shaped teeth at the front of the mouth. You have

eight incisors, four on the upper jaw (two central incisors and two lateral incisors) and four on the lower jaw. Incisors are used for cutting and biting into food.

2. Canines: Canines are the long, pointed teeth located on either side of the incisors. You have four canines, with two in the upper jaw and two in the lower jaw. Canines have a more prominent role in tearing and grasping food.

3. Premolars (bicuspids): Located behind the canines, premolars have a flattened surface with two cusps (points). You should have eight premolars, four in the upper jaw and four in the lower jaw. Premolars assist in chewing and grinding food.

4. Molars: Molars are the largest and strongest teeth located at the back of the mouth. They have a broad, flattened surface with multiple cusps. You usually have twelve molars, including four third molars commonly known

as wisdom teeth. Molars are responsible for crushing, grinding, and chewing food.

Do you know why your molars are shaped like a mountain? Why do they have peaks and valleys? If your teeth were perfectly flat when you were chewing, there would be a lot of force and compression for the teeth to absorb when they came together. How they actually work is the cusps come down into the fossas and the bolus of food escapes out little grooves, thus dissipating the forces. Problems can occur if the posterior teeth are worn down and lack the proper form to chew a bolus of food. Typically, the flatter teeth become, the more horizontally or laterally you move your jaw to chew your food. This lateral or sideways movement puts a lot more wear and stress on the teeth and the jaw joints, just making the teeth that much flatter. Oftentimes, I see the anatomy of molar teeth that are worn. If the tooth needs to be restored, the dentist is in a dilemma, as is usually the case when the opposing tooth is worn as well and there isn't enough space vertically to restore the tooth to the proper anatomy.

Tooth Form Measurements
Posterior

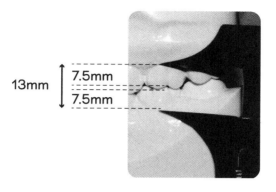

Ideally, you need about 13 mm of space from the gum line of the upper first molar to the gum line of the lower first molar to properly restore the back teeth to the proper anatomy. When there is a lack of space, an interdisciplinary team is needed for reestablishing enough space so that the proper form can be placed back onto the teeth. With the proper form of the back teeth and proper guidance of the front teeth, a more vertical or straight-up-and-down chewing pattern can be realized, saving the teeth from destructive forces. This is why when patients present for treatment and their back teeth are worn down, a discussion needs to occur as to how this problem will be managed. Anterior teeth that are worn can also be a problem. If the front teeth are not long enough to cause the back teeth to separate when the jaw moves, then length will need to be added. But you cannot just add length and form back onto teeth without addressing the underlying cause of why they wore down in the first place. The jaw joints must be in a stable seated position in order to establish a long-term functional occlusion.

Here's a quick explainer of treatment plans and the order of treatment. As discussed, for a complex or interdisciplinary case where an adult has wear on their teeth, the first thing we do is create a list of problems and a treatment plan. Most treatment plans go in this order: first, we have to get the form back on the teeth. If teeth are worn down or flattened, we need to establish proper anatomical form. The second thing we do is straighten them. Next, we work on the bite (discussed in a later chapter) to get the teeth to fit together properly and get the teeth back in their correct position, so to speak. The last thing we do is dial in and get those front teeth exactly where they're supposed to be. Things like airway or a surgical procedure are worked into the treatment plan when necessary. But the main point here is that we get the form on the teeth first.

I see a lot of patients who come in and are unhappy about their teeth. They want an aesthetic improvement. Sometimes they think the problem is they need their teeth straightened, but their underlying problem is they lack the proper form on their teeth for aesthetics and function. You can have nice, straight teeth and still have many things wrong: an open bite, jaw joint out of the socket, etc. Returning to my point earlier in the book about do-it-yourself straightening companies, straight teeth do not necessarily indicate a healthy mouth.

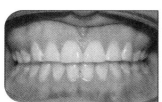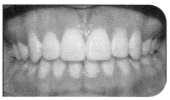

The general dentist restores the form prior to comprehensive orthodontic treatment.

If a patient went to a dentist and stated, "my teeth are getting shorter; why is that?" the dentist would likely ascribe it to grinding and prescribe them a nightguard. Nightguards are great: they help protect the teeth when you sleep and are very effective. But they do not address the underlying problem. It's just a Band-Aid.

Another common misconception is that all of our front teeth should be the same length and height, but that's not how mother nature intended things to be. Your central incisors, the teeth right in front, should be longer than the teeth next to them and proportional in height and width. Unlike a person with extreme wear, they should also have rounded corners. The lateral incisors next to the centrals should be slightly shorter and more rounded. This allows space for the lower canines to slide by without contact.

Our central incisors should be about 12 mm long, and our lower incisors are about 10 mm in length. They should overlap vertically, as we've seen, by about 4 mm. This overlap should be enough to cause separation of the second molars during function. Thus, if the upper central incisor is 12 mm in length and the lower central incisor is 10 mm in length, with 4 mm of vertical overlap, then the distance from the top of the upper central incisor to the bottom of the lower central incisor would be 18 mm. This is a guideline measurement we commonly use when having to restore both upper and lower anterior teeth. The upper canines should also be about 12 mm in length and on the same horizontal plane as the central incisors.

Tooth Form Measurements
Anterior

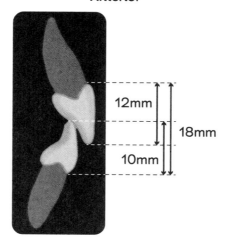

The problem that I feel is most often overlooked by orthodontists is tooth-size discrepancies of upper lateral incisors. The majority of patients have upper lateral incisors that are not wide enough to occupy all of the width that is required in the upper arch to get the upper teeth to fit together properly with the lower teeth. As a result, if all the space is closed, the upper canines end up in a position too far forward to match with the lower teeth. This then becomes a functional problem. The solution is to carefully measure all of the teeth prior to treatment to determine the extent of the tooth-size discrepancy. A simple formula estimates that the width of the lower six front teeth should be 75 percent of the width of the upper six front teeth. To resolve a tooth-size discrepancy, the two most common treatment options are either removing a slight amount of tooth structure in between the lower front teeth or adding to the width of the upper lateral incisors. Typically, most patients elect to have bonding done to establish the proper size of the upper laterals. This not only establishes the ideal position for function but has the added benefit of aesthetic improvement, as they are more proportional in size to the adjacent teeth.

Correction of Tooth Size Discrepancy

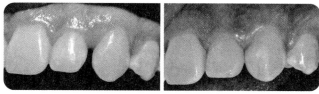

BEFORE   AFTER

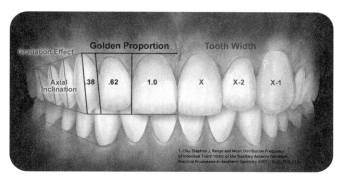

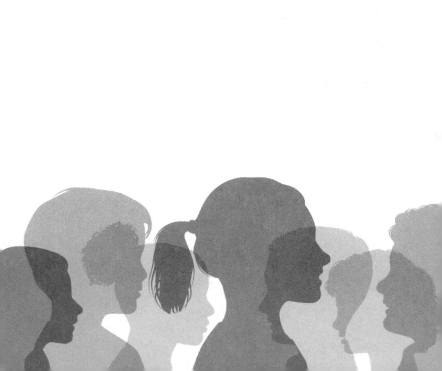

CHAPTER 4

Jaws That Function & a Good Bite

The first principle of FACE orthodontics is proper joint function. There are a few things that set this kind of orthodontic philosophy apart from the rest, and this is chief among them. God made the jaw joint, and he made it to fit into the socket. That's just the way humans are supposed to be. Everything works optimally when this is the case. So, whenever we evaluate bites, we always make sure that the jaw is in the socket. Many times, a patient comes in to see me and they have TMJ issues. Their bite might look fairly good upon initial examination. Without further evaluation, I might assume their jaw joint is in the socket. Their teeth may even look like that perfect zipper I mentioned before in principle two. But as my mentor, Dr. Roth, used to say, "Don't be fooled by what you see in the mouth." In other words, the way someone can bite down can fool you because their jaw still might be out of the socket.

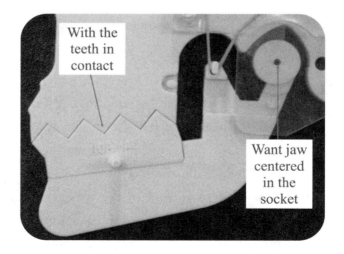

The basic premise is that you have a jaw joint and a jawbone (mandible) with a condyle, which is the circular end of the bone. That condyle belongs in the joint, in the fossa, to function properly. If you are having any kind of TMJ dysfunction, popping or clicking, pain, headaches, or neckaches, that could definitely be attributed to a problem with the jaw joint and its relationship to not being properly positioned in the socket. If the mandible hinges close and there are interferences in the way the teeth contact, this can cause the mandible to shift or deviate. This deflection in the path of closure is usually not tolerated very well by the muscles and the rest of the system over time. The only way a mandible can shift is when it is displaced out of the socket. That's how this condition comes to be. Patients manipulate their jaw out of the socket to accommodate whatever other tooth interferences they may have.

Here's a patient that came in to see me. They had already been through orthodontic treatment but noticed that the front teeth didn't make contact. Their chief concern was TMJ pain. They'd clearly had level

1 orthodontics and their teeth were straight, yet they still didn't fit together. So here's what they did. To get their teeth together, the patient actually used their muscles to shift the jaw out of the socket so the front teeth could contact. This extra amount of movement fatigues the muscles and can also damage the tendons and ligaments of the jaw joint. No wonder they had jaw pain.

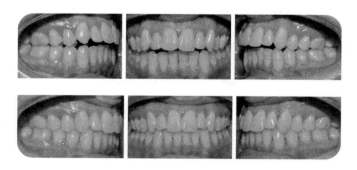

A core principle of the FACE philosophy is to establish a stable, repeatable condylar position. To diagnose if there is a discrepancy in the joint position that might be causing the patient's TMJ pain, we need to see how their bite fits together when their jaw joints are in the socket. To evaluate the relationship of the bite with the jaw joint in the socket, we use an instrument called a jaw-motion simulator (articulator). To do this requires taking a bite registration with soft wax, first of the front teeth and then of the back teeth. The orthodontist carefully monitors the patient upon closing to make sure the patient does not protrude their mandible forward upon closing slowly. When they bite down, we manipulate the jaw so that the jaw joint moves into the socket. Then we either scan or take impressions of their teeth so that models of the teeth can be fabricated. Next, we put the models on the jaw-motion simulator with the wax bite registration in between the upper and lower model. This then shows us how their teeth actually fit together when their jaw joint is in the proper position.

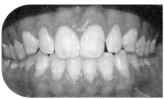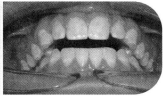

Look at the patient above biting down "normally." Honestly, it's not too bad. The second picture is with their jaw joint actually in the socket. See how bad their bite truly is? You can see how far off it is. I'll repeat, you cannot trust what you see in the mouth. If you truly want to help this patient, and as a health-care provider I certainly do, the best way is to diagnose their bite from a position with their jaw in the socket.

Ensuring the jaw joint is in place when we correct bites and treat patients is a foundational piece of FACE orthodontics.

One of the hard parts of this practice is that it does take an understanding on the patient's part, which is why I'm so glad you picked up this book. It sounds simple, and you may think that all practitioners evaluate their patients' jaw position, but nothing could be further from the truth. It does take more time, but it can prevent so many unrecognized problems from becoming even bigger issues during your course of treatment, not to mention taking a longer period of time in treatment and, in the worst cases, causing there to be a total change in the plan of treatment. This is a simple concept, but it has huge implications. Ensuring the jaw joint is in place when we correct bites and treat patients is a foundational piece of FACE orthodontics.

A Good Bite

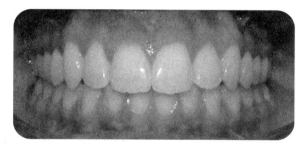

The ideal alignment and relationship of teeth is known as occlusion. In a healthy mouth, the upper and lower teeth should ideally fit together in a way that promotes efficient chewing and minimizes excessive wear or damage. You can take something as thin as a human hair, bite down on it, and be able to tell that there is something between your teeth. The width of a human hair is about one micron or about 1/1,000 of a millimeter. That's how sensitive your proprioception is with your teeth. It doesn't require much of a discrepancy for you to sense something isn't right. It also means that the adjustments we make as orthodontists have to be incredibly precise. When it comes to evaluating a bite, there are several things we consider:

1. Centric Occlusion: This is the natural position where the upper and lower teeth fit together when the jaw is in a relaxed, closed position. The upper teeth slightly overlap the lower teeth vertically and horizontally.

2. Dental Midline: The centerline of the upper teeth should align with the centerline of the lower teeth, ensuring proper symmetry.

3. Contact Points: The teeth should make even contact with each other, allowing for simultaneous chewing and grinding of food. This distribution of force helps prevent excessive wear on specific teeth.

4. Proper Overbite and Overjet: A slight vertical overlap of the upper teeth over the lower teeth (overbite) and a horizontal gap between the upper and lower teeth (overjet) are considered normal and provide proper function.

5. Balanced Occlusion: The forces applied during chewing should be evenly distributed across the teeth, ensuring no undue stress or strain on specific teeth or the jaw joints.

6. Is the mandible free to move without any interferences during function?

That, in a nutshell, makes for a good bite.

I like to think of the bites of the human population as falling into a bell-shaped curve. A small percentage of the population is incredibly sensitive to their bite being off, in the same way that some people are super sensitive to smells or sounds. Unless their bite is right on, they are going to have problems. Treating these patients is hard and requires a special set of skills. On the other end of the bell curve, another small percentage of the population could have a terrible bite but might not ever have any symptoms. Their teeth could wear out or be lost, but they typically don't have any complaints. The majority of us are somewhere in the middle. If the teeth have a significant discrepancy, then sooner or later we are going to experience signs or symptoms. These might include teeth shifting, tooth wear, gum recession, TMJ discomfort, or sensitive teeth. Unfortunately, most adolescents when they finish treatment are not able to determine if their bite fits together properly or not. Hopefully, reading this book will give you the knowledge and understanding of how a bite should fit together.

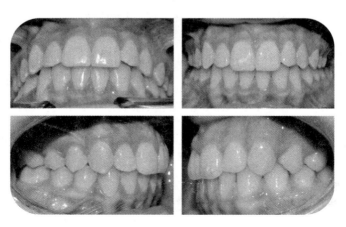

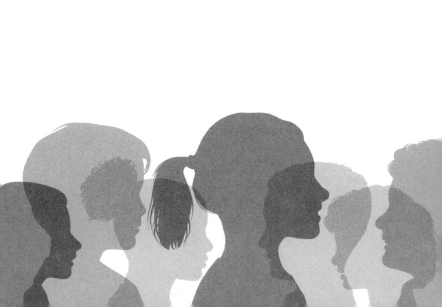

CHAPTER 5

An Open Airway

Diagnosing airway obstructions typically involves a comprehensive evaluation by a healthcare professional, such as an otolaryngologist (ear, nose, and throat specialist) or a sleep medicine specialist. Here are some common steps involved in the diagnosis:

1. Medical History: The healthcare provider will begin by taking a detailed medical history, which includes asking questions about symptoms, previous medical conditions, allergies, and any relevant family history.

2. Physical Examination: A physical examination will be conducted, focusing on the head, neck, and airway. The provider may inspect the nasal passages, throat, tonsils, and adenoids for signs of inflammation, swelling, or structural abnormalities.

3. Imaging Studies: Depending on the suspected cause of the airway obstruction, various imaging studies may be ordered. These can include X-rays, computed tomography (CT) scans, or magnetic resonance imaging (MRI) scans to assess the structures of the airway and identify any blockages or abnormalities.

4. Sleep Studies: In cases where airway obstruction is suspected during sleep, a sleep study, also known as polysomnography, may be conducted. This test monitors various parameters during sleep, including breathing patterns, oxygen levels, and brain activity, to diagnose sleep-related breathing disorders such as sleep apnea.

5. Additional Tests: Additional tests may be performed based on the specific situation. These can include allergy testing, lung function tests, or endoscopic examinations to visualize the airway in more detail.

With the introduction of cone-beam technology into orthodontics, evaluation of airway constrictions and anomalies has become easier to uncover and diagnose. Obstructive sleep-disordered breathing (OSDB) is not diagnosed with imaging, but imaging can identify patients with airways that are at risk for obstruction and other anatomic characteristics that may contribute to OSDB. The airway extending from the tip of the nose to the superior end of the trachea can be visualized on cone-beam computed tomography (CBCT) scans. Because these scans also include the jaws, teeth, cranial base, spine, and facial soft tissues, there is an opportunity to evaluate the functional and developmental relationships between these structures.

The skeletal support for your airway is provided by the cranial base (superiorly), spine (posteriorly), nasal septum (anterosuperiorly), jaws, and hyoid bone (anteriorly). The airway valves include the soft palate, tongue, and epiglottis. Airway obstructions or encroachments are of interest because they increase airway resistance and may contribute to obstructive sleep-disordered breathing (OSDB). So, visualization and calculation of the airway dimensions are important. Some of the most common encroachments include turbinates; adenoids; a long, soft palate; an enlarged tongue; and pharyngeal and lingual tonsils. Some less-common ones are polyps and tumors. As a precaution, I'd recommend having your cone-beam radiograph reviewed by a radiologist. They can provide a 3D volumetric study of your airway and surrounding structures. Dr. David Hatcher is a maxillofacial radiologist, founder of BeamReaders, and a leader and pioneer in interpreting CBCT scans. Dr. Hatcher has recommended the following dimensions as a guideline in assisting in determining the probability a patient may have severe obstructive sleep apnea (OSA):

- High probability of severe OSA: < 52 mm^2

- Intermediate probability of severe OSA: 52–110 mm^2

- Low probability of severe OSA: > 110 mm^2

Depending on the location of the narrowing, a referral may be required. Constrictions caused by adenoids and tonsils will require an evaluation by an ENT. An underlying skeletal discrepancy might involve an oral and maxillofacial surgeon to evaluate if the upper and/or lower jaw is in a retruded position. Impingements caused by the tongue or palate can oftentimes be improved by orthodontics. So, being able to properly locate where and what is causing a constriction in the airway will determine who might be best equipped to assist in treatment. Understand that not all breathing issues are related to just the size of the airway. I've seen patients with large airways who suffer from severe sleep apnea, but they are the exception. Research has proven that there is a direct correlation between the size of someone's airway and their symptoms. A sleep study still remains the gold standard in diagnosing sleep apnea.

Look at the image below. Do you see the constriction? It's where that little white circle is, and I can tell you right now it's likely due to enlarged adenoids. For that, we refer out to an ENT. We also often see constrictions due to an enlarged tongue. Or perhaps the tongue is of normal size, but due to the width of the palate, there isn't enough room. Sometimes the lower jaw is too far back and is compressing the tongue.

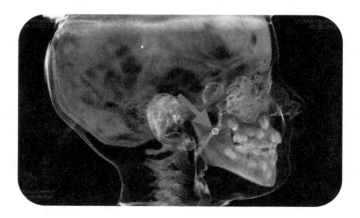

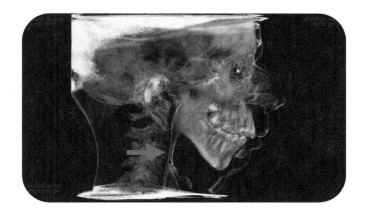

Let's look at some examples. Here's a classic example of the lower jaw being too far back. This retruded jaw is compressing against the airway. You can see that the upper part of the airway looks to be of normal width, as the constriction is down more in the throat. Notice how the jaw angulation is quite steep. In general, if there is a problem with the tongue or jaw, the ENT isn't able to help these patients at all other than recommend a continuous positive airway pressure machine (CPAP).

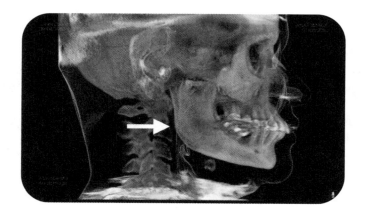

In this case, if you look at this patient's tongue, you can even see what we refer to as scalloping, the little indentations along the edge of the tongue, due to the tongue pushing against the teeth. The pressure of the tongue against the teeth actually moves the teeth forward, thus affecting the bite and function. The tongue is being directed to move forward in order to open the airway. If the tongue can't find enough space by pushing everything forward, the only place for it to rest is in the back of the throat. Look at her airway dimension. It's 17.8. Remember, for an adult, it should be 150, and under 54 is a severe risk for sleep apnea. This becomes a dilemma for both the patient and the orthodontist.

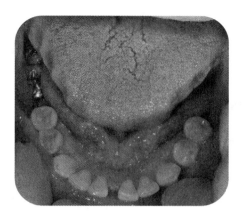

Of course, I can close the spacing. I could put enough force on those teeth to close them. But as soon as we remove those forces, they'll go right back, because we haven't solved the underlying problem. Actually, with her teeth straightened, her tongue would have even less

Often, patients come for aesthetic concerns, but there are many more underlying problems we discover.

space, and her breathing might actually get worse. I wouldn't be doing her a favor at all. Her real problem is the enlarged tongue. Treatment-wise, she has a couple of options. She could opt for jaw surgery to move both upper or lower jaws forward or undergo a procedure to actually make the tongue smaller. It's always best to educate patients as to what their options are and let them make informed decisions. Sometimes doing what might not be the easiest turns out to be what is best for an improved quality of life.

Often, patients come for aesthetic concerns, but there are many more underlying problems we discover. While you can make a good guess about someone's airway by looking at it, there is always a chance that you have misjudged. I've seen normal-sized people with perfect profiles have a constriction, and I've seen overweight people with a retruded chin have a great airway. You cannot judge a book by its cover, which is why we rely on a CBCT to screen everyone.

It's important to note that orthodontic treatment alone may not be sufficient to address severe airway obstructions or conditions like sleep apnea. In such cases, a multidisciplinary approach involving various medical interventions may be necessary. It's crucial to consult with healthcare professionals specializing in airway disorders to determine the most appropriate treatment plan for individual cases.

Again, the definitive diagnosis for OSDB is a sleep study, which is the gold standard. Thus, the only definitive way to determine whether or not someone truly has sleep apnea is to do an overnight sleep study. Brain activity can be evaluated to determine what levels of sleep the patient experiences. Breathing and heart rate are recorded as well. Apnea episodes (when someone stops breathing for longer than ten seconds) are measured. The following scale is used to categorize the severity of someone's sleep apnea:

None/Normal	AHI is < 5 per hour
Mild	AHI is ≥ 5 per hour, but < 15 per hour
Moderate	AHI is ≥ 15 per hour, but < 30 per hour
Severe	AHI is ≥ 30 per hour

There are also at-home studies that patients can use. Even just a Fitbit that you wear all night can give you some pretty good data on the quality of your sleep. These devices cannot, however, measure the levels of your sleep since they do not measure brain activity.

Airway Concerns in Children

A recent study found that 50 percent of children with ADHD had signs of sleep-disordered breathing compared to only 22 percent of children without ADHD. In other words, there's a strong link between kids that have ADHD and the quality of sleep they're getting. Another study found a similar correlation with restless leg syndrome.[1]

---

1   Ritesh Kalaskar, Priyanka Bhaje, Ashita Kalaskar, and Abhijeet Faye, "Sleep Difficulties and Symptoms of Attention-Deficit Hyperactivity Disorder in Children with Mouth Breathing," *International Journal of Clinical Pediatric Dentistry* 14, no. 5 (Sept.–Oct. 2021): 604–9, https://doi.org/10.5005%2Fjp-journals-10005-1987.

One of the main focuses of my practice is treating sleep disorders in children. If a mother comes in and mentions that her child snores, that's a huge red flag. You do not want to put that off or avoid it. Children need sleep much, much more than adults for the development of their brains and body, so losing sleep is detrimental. Here are some things to look for in your child:

- Your child is breathing or just sitting at the table with their mouth open. They don't have their lips closed and are breathing through their mouth. I could fill a whole other book with things that are bad about mouth-breathing. Look for chapped lips or inflamed, red gums.

- Bags under their eyes. This is called venous pooling. It looks like raccoon eyes.

- Head posture. Your child's neck is extended, and they look like they're constantly looking up. They do this to try and enlarge their airway.

- Any kind of hearing loss.

- Head and neck pain, often from improper posture.

- Fatigue first thing in the morning.

If your child exhibits any of these regularly, you should seek care. Early intervention is critical, and so is good-quality sleep. Any of these signs could mean that your child has a constricted airway, and left untreated, it will only get worse.

Sleep-disordered breathing (SDB) in children can be treated by orthodontics through various methods aimed at improving the airway and addressing the underlying causes of the breathing difficulties. Here are some common orthodontic treatments for SDB in children:

1. Rapid Palatal Expansion (RPE): Narrow dental arches can contribute to airway obstruction. RPE is a technique that uses an orthodontic appliance to gradually widen the upper jaw and increase the available space for

the tongue. This can help alleviate breathing difficulties by improving the airway passage.

2. Mandibular Advancement Devices (MADs): MADs are removable appliances that are custom-made to fit over the teeth and reposition the lower jaw slightly forward. By advancing the mandible, MADs help to open the airway, reducing the severity of breathing problems during sleep.

3. Functional Appliances: Functional appliances are orthodontic devices that work by influencing the growth and position of the jaws. These appliances can help address skeletal imbalances, improve the alignment of the jaws, and consequently enhance the airway.

4. Orthodontic Tooth Movement: In some cases, orthodontic tooth movement can be utilized to optimize the alignment of the teeth and jaws, thereby creating more space

within the oral cavity and improving the airway passage.

5. Myofunctional Therapy: Myofunctional exercises aim to strengthen the muscles of the tongue, lips, and face, improving tongue posture, swallowing patterns, and overall muscle function. This can contribute to better airway function and reduce breathing difficulties.

6. Collaborative Treatment: Working in collaboration with other healthcare professionals such as otolaryngologists, sleep medicine specialists, or pediatric dentists to develop comprehensive treatment plans for children with SDB is quite common. This multidisciplinary approach ensures that the child's condition is assessed comprehensively, and the most appropriate treatment options are chosen based on the specific needs of the child.

It's important to note that the appropriate treatment for SDB in children depends on the specific diagnosis and severity of the condition. Each child's case is unique, and the treatment plan will be tailored to their individual needs.

Other Good Oral Health Habits

We now know that when we start to see signs of crooked teeth, it usually means the jaws aren't growing properly. Bad oral habits, like not swallowing the right way and breathing through your mouth, are also causes of crooked teeth and jaws. The forces of the tongue, cheeks, and lips combined with these bad oral habits can have a big effect on how your teeth are positioned. A normal top jaw grows properly because the tongue rests in the correct position, which is in the roof of your mouth, appropriately known as the correct tongue-resting position. If your tongue rests in the floor of the mouth, then the tongue does not maintain an outward pressure against the upper teeth, and the inward forces of the cheeks then begin to constrict the upper arch. This then can cause additional problems with crowding and a discrepancy in how the upper and lower teeth fit together.

Another thing to watch out for is if you're swallowing the wrong way, with lots of movement in the bottom lip. Yes, there is a right and wrong way to swallow. When you swallow incorrectly, your front teeth will be pushed backward. This also causes your teeth to be crowded. Here's a quick recap of things to do to help maintain a clear airway, good bite, and straight teeth. These are twice as important to watch out for in children as they are in adults.

- Have the tongue rest in the roof of your mouth.

- Breathe through your nose.

- Close your mouth when you breathe.

- Swallow properly.

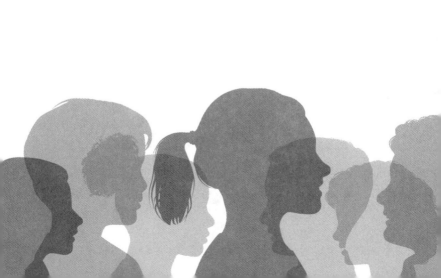

CHAPTER 6

Interceptive Treatment

Interceptive orthodontic treatment, also known as early orthodontic treatment, is a proactive approach that aims to address certain orthodontic issues in children at an early age. The goal of interceptive treatment is to guide the growth and development of the jaws and teeth, correct specific problems, and prevent potential complications from worsening in the future. Here are some common aspects and techniques involved in interceptive orthodontic treatment for children:

1. Evaluation and Assessment: First a thorough evaluation of the child's dental and facial structures is done. This may involve taking a scan of the teeth, CBCT X-ray, photographs, and conducting a clinical examination. The child's dental alignment and jaw relationship will be assessed, and then any issues that may require early intervention will be discussed.

2. Space Maintenance/Regaining: Interceptive orthodontics may involve creating or maintaining space in the dental arches to accommodate permanent teeth. If a primary tooth is lost prematurely due to decay or extraction, a space maintainer may be used to prevent neighboring teeth from shifting into the empty space and blocking the eruption path of permanent teeth.

3. Guiding Jaw Growth: In cases where jaw growth discrepancies are detected, interceptive treatment may include techniques to guide and influence the growth of the jaws.

Functional appliances, such as expanders or activators, may be used to stimulate or modify the growth of the upper or lower jaw, improving their alignment and relationship.

4. Correcting Malocclusions: Interceptive orthodontic treatment can address specific malocclusions, such as crossbites, open bites, or deep bites. Functional appliances, orthodontic braces, or other removable appliances may be employed to guide tooth movement and correct the bite relationship.

5. Addressing Habits: Interceptive treatment may also involve addressing harmful oral habits that can affect dental and facial development. Thumb sucking, tongue thrusting, or prolonged pacifier use can cause misalignment of teeth or jaw growth issues. We may provide guidance and strategies to help the child break these habits.

6. Monitoring Growth and Development: During interceptive treatment, regular

follow-up appointments are scheduled to monitor the child's growth and dental changes. This allows us to assess treatment progress, make necessary adjustments, and ensure that the child's dental and skeletal development is on track.

It's important to note that not all children require interceptive orthodontic treatment. The decision to pursue early intervention depends on the individual child's orthodontic needs and the severity of the identified issues. Early treatment can often simplify or minimize the need for comprehensive orthodontic treatment in the future, improving the child's oral health and overall facial aesthetics.

The American Association of Orthodontists recommends children have their first visit to an orthodontist by age seven. I agree with them and would add that it's never too early if you detect a problem.

This chapter is about different types of dental issues that arise from having a mixture of baby teeth and permanent teeth. So, obviously, we're talking about children and adolescents. I have mentioned many of the problems in this chapter before, but here the focus is on how they affect children and what options are available for early intervention. This is a particularly important chapter for parents, as these problems can be solved most easily in childhood.

Let's first look at tongue ties. It is estimated that between 4 and 10 percent of the population is afflicted. One thing we need to be on the lookout for in infants is tongue ties. This is when a piece of the tongue called the frenum is attached to the floor of the mouth. This can limit babies early in life, making breastfeeding nearly impossible for both the infant and the mother. Babies with a tongue tie will often have a poor latch, whether breastfed or bottle-fed. This poor latch can result in your baby taking in excess air, which then sits in their stomach. This results in colic-like symptoms of crying, pulling up knees, and bloating. However, not all tongue ties are diagnosed at this time and can eventually interfere with the ability to make certain sounds—such as "t," "d," "z," "s," "th," "r," and "l." A tongue tie can also make it more difficult for one to clean food from around the teeth and the back of the mouth, thus leading to poorer hygiene and a greater chance of cavities and periodontal disease.

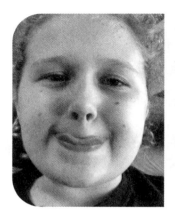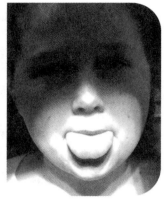

Typically, treatment can be provided in babies younger than three months old using a topical anesthetic and laser. Because the area has few nerve endings or blood vessels, local anesthetic is usually not required. A laser vaporizes the tissue, making healing quick and easy. Post-op, the difference in function is dramatic. This simple, quick procedure (usually less than a minute) is done as an outpatient procedure.

Here are some signs to be aware of if you suspect that your baby may have a tongue tie:

- Can't latch well

- Tends to chew more than suck

- Poor weight gain

- Feeds for a long time, takes a short break, then feeds for another long stretch

- Is fussy when trying to feed

- Makes a clicking sound while feeding

- Seems hungry all the time

Remember the equilibrium I talked about between the tongue and cheeks? Your cheeks press inward, and your tongue maintains that outward pressure. If someone is tongue-tied, they potentially cannot rest their tongue high enough in the palate, or the roof of the mouth. You'll remember from the last chapter that this is exactly where we want the tongue to rest. If the tongue isn't resting in the top of the mouth to maintain the width of the palate, the inward pressure from the cheeks will cause a constriction of the palate. This is one of the main reasons for a crossbite, where upper teeth fit inside the lower teeth.

Most people had no idea their tongue and cheeks were working so hard, even when at rest.

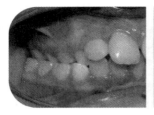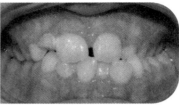

Posterior crossbites can develop on either or both sides. If untreated, a unilateral crossbite can lead to uneven mandibular growth and facial asymmetry. Typically, kids will have to shift their jaw to get their teeth to come together. Of course, anytime you shift your jaw, that pulls your jaw joints out of the socket, creating a whole host of cyclical problems. You also see the more common dental issues, like TMJ, neck and jaw pain, etc., with crossbites. If your child has a crossbite, like approximately 10 percent of kids, you need to seek treatment once discovered; delaying treatment can lead to additional skeletal issues. Palatal expansion can also provide relief of some breathing problems by increasing the volume of the nasal airway and providing more tongue space. Expansion can assist in redirecting growth and development—thus significantly reducing the number of extractions, which assists in creating bigger, broader arch smiles.

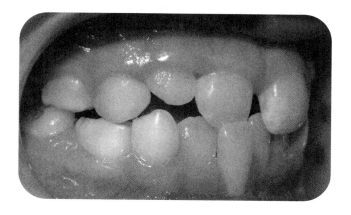

Crossbites associated with the front teeth are known as anterior crossbites. The two most common causes of anterior crossbites are crowding and a skeletal growth imbalance. The thing we worry about with a crossbite of the front teeth is that if the top teeth aren't out in front and instead rest behind the lower teeth, they start pushing the lower teeth forward. Every time the child bites down, it puts forward pressure on the lower front teeth, which can lead to the gum tissue receding. If a gum graft were done (a simple surgery where you transplant gum from the roof of the mouth to the area of recession), I doubt it would be maintained unless the crossbite were corrected to relieve the pressure of the upper teeth pushing the lower teeth forward.

Crossbites are far and away the most common problem we see in children. I cannot emphasize enough that these should be corrected as soon as possible. The longer you wait to correct a crossbite, the more problems it will cause. Gum recession is a big one, and tooth wear is another. And that wear is always going to be there. Even if we correct the crossbite later, the teeth still aren't going to look as nice as they possibly could.

Let's look a little closer at some of the consequences here for children. An overjet means that there is a horizontal discrepancy between the position of the top teeth and bottom teeth: think of protruded upper-front teeth. It's commonly known as an overbite, but since you've read a book about orthodontics, you know better. Usually, it's a problem with the lower jaw being too far back, known as mandibular retrusion. But it can also be that the upper teeth are too far forward. What we worry about here is when the back teeth don't fit together the way they should, they're going to be hitting end to end, causing wear. We don't care about this so much in baby teeth. They're going to lose those. But if this occurs with the six-year molars, that's a problem.

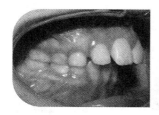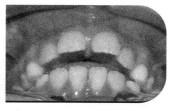

It won't surprise you to know that a common dental incident in kids with an overjet is trauma to the upper teeth. I see at least one or two kids every summer that are running around a swimming pool, slip and fall, or get hit in the face with a baseball and fracture one or both of their protruded front teeth.

When your teeth are too far forward, they're more at risk for trauma.

I've also noticed that among children whose lower jaw is too far back, at around age ten they will begin to notice it themselves and subconsciously push their jaw forward because they realize it doesn't look good and they become self-conscious. They may also be posturing their jaw forward or tipping their head back in order to open their airway further. Even though this may be pulling the jaw out of the socket or causing neck discomfort, the body's need for oxygen supersedes all else.

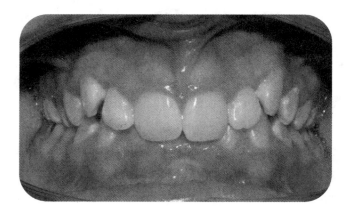

Let's discuss deep bites, also known as a deep overbite. Deep bites are very common, affecting as many as one in five patients seeking orthodontic treatment. When you have an excessive vertical overlap of the front top teeth with the bottom front teeth, it is referred to as a deep bite. The most serious problem associated with a deep bite is wear on the lower front teeth. This is due to the movement of the lower jaw upon opening and closing. There isn't the proper clearance for the teeth to avoid excessive contact, and thus it leads to tooth wear. Sometimes the upper teeth are tipped inward, which only worsens the problem. If there is a significant skeletal discrepancy, the lower teeth will often contact the palatal tissue just behind the upper-front teeth, causing trauma to the palatal tissue. This can be quite painful.

So, the opposite of a deep bite is an open bite. With open bites, there is a lack of vertical overlap of the front teeth. It can be due to an underlying skeletal problem, enlarged adenoids, or airway obstruction, but is most commonly caused by a thumb/finger-sucking habit. Even if you stop the thumb/finger habit, often the tongue will maintain the open bite. This is because if you try to swallow with your mouth open, you will take your tongue and put it between your teeth to swallow. Try it now. You need to create a seal in the anterior to effectively swallow, and you can't do it with your mouth open or teeth apart. The tongue maintains the anterior open bite. If you can catch these early in children, often all it takes is an appliance to correct. Appliances keep the tongue back so the teeth can erupt and grow down.

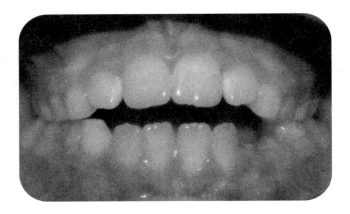

Treating these open bites as an adult or late teen can be rather difficult because teeth tend to lose their ability to erupt after childhood. This is why appliances in adults are noneffective for the most part. Open bites can lead to several different problems. First, as mentioned previously in this book, the anterior teeth need to overlap in order to guide the movement of the lower jaw during the chewing process. Anterior contact prevents the back teeth from touching during movement. Thus, lack of proper anterior guidance allows the back teeth to contact during lateral movements, which typically results in tooth wear. Also, there is a correlation between anterior open bites and TMJ pain.

Other side effects associated with anterior open bites include difficulty chewing and incising food. Just imagine biting into a sandwich and the lettuce doesn't get shredded but instead hangs out of the front of your mouth. Remember also how the tips of the upper teeth are supposed to follow the curvature of the lower lip. Typically, patients with anterior open bites have just the opposite: their back teeth are down farther than their front teeth. This can give the appearance of a gummy smile in the posterior. In some situations, their upper-front teeth barely show when smiling. Speech can also be a problem, as some people will have a lisp.

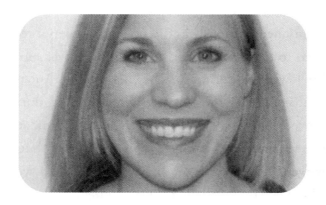

Posterior open bites are not as common as anterior open bites but most commonly develop due to ankylosed teeth (teeth fused to the bone, which inhibits their vertical growth). Any ankylosed tooth should be removed as soon as possible to avoid over-eruption of the teeth in the opposing arch. In

Teeth will drift to wherever there is space, up or down, forward, or back.

these cases, retainers and/or space maintainers are needed to prevent unwanted tooth movement. Teeth might also need to be removed early due to decay or trauma. Once again, proper planning is required based on age, development, type of malocclusion, etc., to determine the proper form of retention. Permanent teeth erupt based on the amount of root formation they have. They do not erupt any earlier just because a baby tooth falls out or is removed early. Space maintainers ensure that the baby teeth do not drift over into the space reserved for the permanent tooth. That could cause the entire midline to drift toward the side where the space is, throwing off arch symmetry. Teeth will drift to wherever there is space, up or down, forward, or back.

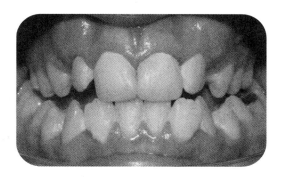

Let's talk about crowding. Typically, when we see a permanent tooth that is blocked out, again we'll see shifting of the midline, creating an improper bite. The teeth don't fit together because one tooth is totally blocked out and everything has shifted around. The thing parents don't like about this (or children either) is that it's unaesthetic. This is why, if kids are evaluated at an early age, we can expand and develop those arches and make enough space for all of the teeth to fit.

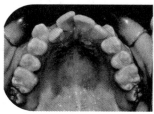 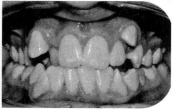

Look at the patient below. Those two pictures are of the same person. Notice the change in the arch form, going from a V shape to a nice big U. The V is narrow and constricted, blocking out the teeth. The U nicely allows for all the teeth. But you could not do this easily for an adult. Expanding a palate is much easier in a child. And most of these expansions only require a few months, but the window is short. That's why early intervention is critical.

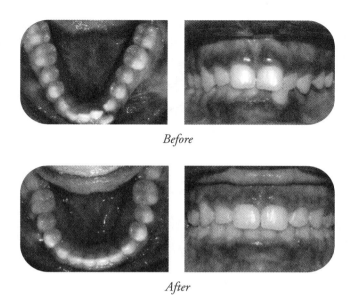

Before

After

The fixes for so many of these problems are quick, simple, and easy if caught early. Many times we don't even need to take a mold or do anything that gags the child. We just use a digital scanner and order their appliance, which is fabricated in a lab. In many cases, these early solutions make the second phase of treatment, after all their permanent teeth are in, quicker and easier as well.

CHAPTER 7

Interdisciplinary Treatment

Interdisciplinary orthodontic treatment, also known as multidisciplinary orthodontic treatment, refers to a collaborative approach involving multiple health-care professionals from different specialties to address complex dental and facial issues comprehensively. This approach recognizes that certain orthodontic problems may be influenced by or have an impact on other areas of oral health or overall well-being. Here's an overview of interdisciplinary orthodontic treatment:

1. Initial Assessment: The process begins with a comprehensive evaluation to assess the patient's dental and facial structures, malocclusions, and potential orthodontic treatment needs. The orthodontist identifies any complex issues that may require input from other specialists.

2. Treatment Planning: Based on the assessment, the orthodontist works in collaboration with other healthcare professionals to develop an integrated treatment plan. The team may include specialists such as oral and maxillofacial surgeons, periodontists, prosthodontists, endodontists, otolaryngologists, speech therapists, and others, depending on the specific needs of the patient.

3. Orthodontic Treatment: The orthodontist takes the lead in providing orthodontic treatment, which may involve using braces, aligners, or other orthodontic appliances to correct dental and skeletal alignment issues.

The orthodontist may also address specific concerns related to the occlusion (bite) and alignment of the teeth.

4. Collaborative Interventions: Depending on the complexity of the case, other specialists may provide concurrent or subsequent treatments to complement orthodontic therapy. Here are some examples:

   A. Oral and Maxillofacial Surgeons: They may perform orthognathic surgery to correct severe jaw discrepancies or extract impacted teeth that hinder orthodontic treatment.

   B. Periodontists: They may address gum diseases, grafting for recession, or bone-grafting procedures to enhance the support and aesthetics around the teeth.

   C. Prosthodontists: They may contribute to restorative or rehabilitative treatments involving dental crowns, bridges, or dental implants to improve function and aesthetics.

D. Endodontists: They may perform root canal treatments to address infected or damaged teeth as part of the overall treatment plan.

E. Otolaryngologists: They may evaluate and treat any underlying airway issues, such as sleep apnea or breathing difficulties, in conjunction with orthodontic interventions.

The combined expertise and collaboration of different specialists allow for a more thorough assessment, customized treatment planning, and improved overall oral health and aesthetics.

Not all malocclusions can be corrected with just orthodontic treatment alone. This is due to underlying skeletal malalignments, excessive tooth wear, bone loss, gingival recession, implant placement, missing teeth, habits, abnormal growth, condylar resorption, endodontic involvement, impacted teeth, and constricted airways.

Simply straightening teeth with orthodontics does not address all the problems patients present with. Thus, to correct these multifactorial problems, an interdisciplinary team is utilized, comprised of different dental and medical specialists who employ their expertise and skills to provide solutions to the various problems that patients present with. The treatment outcome is improved and simplified by utilizing an interdisciplinary-team approach. It works out best for the patient if this team of practitioners shares a similar treatment philosophy and has previously worked together, so the patient is not hearing contradictory messages from practitioner to practitioner. Each individual practitioner is responsible for providing a piece of the comprehensive treatment plan and making sure that all the problems are addressed to solve even the most complex of dentofacial or skeletal issues.

Adults typically have more problems than kids due to mutilation over the years. Orthodontic treatment for adults has seen rapid growth in recent years due to an increased awareness of the problems associated with a malocclusion and the benefits that come from treatment. Advances in treatment techniques, materials, and aesthetic appliances have made it more appealing for adults to decide to pursue treatment. The goal of this chapter is to share some of the recent advancements to address many of the more common problems we face today.

Interdisciplinary Philosophy & Treatment Planning

It's nice when the entire interdisciplinary team shares the same philosophy (as has been previously outlined in this book). This allows there to be a treatment plan that all the team members can agree upon, which addresses the patient's needs and desires. The most common problem that I see in orthodontics is a lack of properly diagnosing an underlying skeletal problem. The orthodontist thinks they can correct the problem with just conventional orthodontic techniques only to find out three-plus years later that they cannot achieve a good result unless there is a change in the treatment plan. This is an unfortunate situation to end up in. I try to avoid this outcome, even if it means not initiating treatment to begin with.

I understand that not all patients want to undergo the needed procedures to correct all their problems. In these situations, the patient has the option to decide on what they may want, ranging from limited treatment of just straightening the teeth and not correcting the bite to no treatment at all. The situation that no one wants is when a patient enters treatment thinking that they are going to have all their chief concerns corrected along with a functional bite, only to find out months later that their teeth are straight, but their bite or symptoms are now worse. This is not the outcome anyone wants!

The take-home message here is that to correct underlying skeletal problems in orthodontics, it takes more than what conventional braces or aligners by themselves can correct. That is why an interdisciplinary team is required to achieve the result that the patient needs. As tempting as it may be to select a direct-to-consumer product because of costs and ease, buyer beware! Unsupervised orthodontic treatment cannot do the job that may be required to achieve the results that a patient desires.

Arriving at the proper diagnosis and treatment plan is the most crucial of all processes. It is essential for the orthodontist to have as much information available as possible to make the best decisions. These include radiographic imaging, mounted study models, intra-oral and facial photographs, patient examination and history, and the patient's chief concern. Once this information is obtained, the development of a comprehensive treatment plan can be initiated. The orthodontist not only needs to know what their capabilities are, but those of different disciplines in dentistry and medicine.

I find it hard to tell a patient exactly what they need at an initial examination, especially if there are multiple issues to consider. I prefer to have full records taken and evaluated prior to rendering a treatment plan. Time taken in the beginning not only benefits the patient, but having the correct plan of treatment greatly decreases the amount of time that a patient spends in treatment, which is a win-win situation for both the patient and orthodontist.

To solve complex dentofacial problems, I like to break them down in a systematic manner. First, I look at the form of the teeth and ask whether restorative dentistry will be required prior to orthodontics to restore the worn teeth. Also, what is the level of bone and soft-tissue support around the teeth? Is a periodontist going to be required before, during, or after treatment? Is there any resorption of the condyles? If so, then that must be addressed first.

Next, I evaluate what will be required to establish a functional occlusion, and I ask how this will affect the patient's profile and smile aesthetics. Will it require some form of skeletal anchorage or surgery to achieve proper function and balance? An airway evaluation is essential in determining the extent of treatment that may be rendered. I ask the question, "Are you having any issues breathing, sleeping, snoring, etc.?" Many times, patients are experiencing sleep and breathing issues and are unaware that the orthodontic interdisciplinary team can address and correct these problems as well.

Once the full scope of problems and treatment desires is compiled and input from other specialists regarding treatment are evaluated, then an ideal, realistic plan of treatment that addresses the problem list and the patient's chief complaint is formulated. Each problem on the problem list needs to be addressed. Alternative treatment plans are developed to provide the patient with options based on what their chief concern might be.

As an orthodontist, it is beneficial to utilize a computerized treatment-planning software program so the patient can visualize the treatment outcome. This can assist the patient in seeing not only their teeth but any changes in their soft-tissue profile. There are several things the patient must consider, including costs, risks, and benefits. Overall, the team wants to maximize treatment results for the patient with minimal invasiveness and with satisfaction of the patient's desires. It is essential that each of the interdisciplinary team members understands their responsibility in the plan of treatment.

To assure a smooth flow throughout the treatment process, it is a benefit to have an organized, written plan of treatment with sequencing as to what and when each step of treatment is scheduled to occur. This is a great service for the patient, allowing them to plan their schedule and finances accordingly. FACE orthodontics always comes back to the goals set at the beginning of treatment. The closer we can come to achieving those goals,

FACE orthodontics always comes back to the goals set at the beginning of treatment.

the better long-term stability and health the patient is going to enjoy.

One of the limiting factors in orthodontic movement is the availability of bone and gingival tissue surrounding the teeth. Teeth that are in improper positions often have gingival recession and periodontal breakdown. Maintenance of periodontal health is a key focus to everyone on the interdisciplinary team. Properly positioned teeth allow much easier access to improve hygiene. Orthodontic treatment can greatly enhance the long-term prognosis of teeth with compromised positions by relocating them into areas of more adequate bone support.

Treatment Alternatives:

SFOT

Limitations in traditional orthodontic movement and the time it takes is a deterrent to the desires of today's patient. In situations where the amount of bone is limited and the teeth need to be better positioned, a procedure known as surgically facilitated orthodontic tooth movement (SFOT), can be most beneficial in correcting malocclusion and enhancing the bone around the teeth.

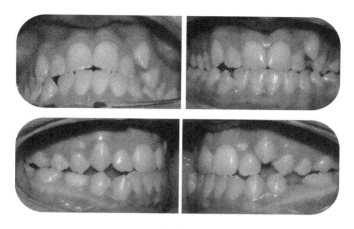

Before

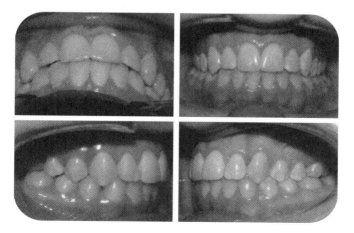

After

The concept of facilitating orthodontic tooth movement was proposed over one hundred years ago. Being able to take advantage of tissue engineering has allowed the interdisciplinary team to now modify alveolar bone to not only shorten treatment times but to expand the scope of possible tooth movement, which in the past was only correctable with much more invasive surgical procedures.

This is performed in a surgeon's office as an outpatient procedure. Done under sedation, narrow vertical incisions between the roots of the upper teeth are performed. In addition, bone-grafting material is placed to enhance the thickness of supporting bone. Surgically facilitated procedures are generally more stable, have fewer complications and reduced costs, and are more predictable than orthognathic surgery. Normal healing occurs through a cascade of molecular and cellular events triggered in response to injury. The process of surgically facilitated rapid tooth movement is like that of normal fracture healing of a bone, and there are several phases, including a reactive, reparative, and a remodeling phase.

I have found this to be a most beneficial procedure for patients with an underbite tendency due to a lack of upper-jaw growth and to resolve severe crowding. Class III malocclusions originating from excessive mandibular growth in growing patients are not good candidates, and in most cases, orthognathic surgery will be recommended after the end of growth.

TEMPORARY ANCHORAGE

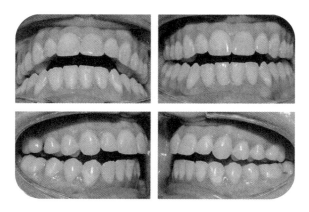

Before

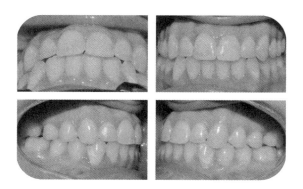

After

The placement of a screw into the bone, subsequently removed after treatment, for the use of anchorage to move teeth, has been gaining a great amount of popularity in a short amount of time and for good reason. It has all but replaced headgear to reposition the posterior molars for bite correction. In addition, temporary appliances that are secured with small titanium screws are also being used for expansion, distalization, and just about any movement that might be needed, everything from expansion of the maxilla to correction of an overjet to anterior open-bite closure and even intrusion of teeth into the bone.

Temporary appliances have proven to be a very predictable, noninvasive, and cost-effective means to achieve tooth alignment and bite correction that in the past would have only been achievable with either extraction of permanent teeth or once again, more invasive surgical procedures.

ORTHOGNATHIC SURGERY

I was very fortunate that while I was an orthodontic resident, I met Dr. Bill Arnett, an oral and maxillofacial surgeon from Santa Barbara, California. His mentorship and guidance regarding how to properly evaluate and create treatment plans for patients with skeletal discrepancies has been one of the greatest blessings of my career. His philosophy of treatment goes hand in hand with that of the FACE orthodontic philosophy. Dr. Arnett teaches a philosophy known as face, airway, and bite (FAB).

Unfortunately, if a malocclusion is due to an underlying skeletal discrepancy, then it cannot be treated with orthodontics alone. Orthognathic surgery may be the best overall treatment option to address all the problems and achieve the best outcome. As my orthodontic mentor, Dr. Ron Roth, would say, "Orthodontics became a lot easier when I stopped trying to correct the things I couldn't change due to skeletal problems."

I have seen countless situations throughout my career where patients have been in orthodontic treatment for years trying to achieve an acceptable result only to end up many times in situations worse than when they started. Hygiene issues, tooth decay, root resorption, periodontal recession, tooth wear, TMJ discomfort, and orthodontic relapse are just a few of the problems associated with trying to correct skeletal problems with orthodontics alone.

Orthognathic surgery to correct severe deformities has improved greatly due to innovations in the biomaterials used and the advanced technology now being utilized to virtually plan surgery. Today's 3D virtual planning allows visualization of both before- and after-surgery prediction. The cone-beam X-ray is used to precisely position both the upper and lower jaw, taking into consideration any facial discrepancies, cants, asymmetries, as well as airway constrictions. Custom-manufactured titanium plates and screws are used to hold the jaws in their new positions while the healing occurs. This allows patients to not only recover much faster than before, but the surgical positioning of the jaws is precisely where planned. No longer are patients wired closed, which besides being uncomfortable was unstable as well.

Remember that not all orthodontists receive extensive training in surgical orthodontics, and not all oral surgeons are up on the latest techniques. Orthognathic surgery isn't something that you want to go through twice; thus, it is advisable to seek treatment with an orthodontist and surgeon who have a good and frequent working relationship. Like anything else, the more you do something the better and more efficient you become.

In addition to functional problems, some elect to have a surgical procedure based on facial aesthetics. Typically, patients with a prominent lower jaw tend to be more self-conscious and rate themselves as less attractive than those patients who have a retrusive profile. Thus, aesthetic improvement is the biggest motivating factor for undergoing treatment. Other problems, such as speech, TMJ, sleep apnea, difficulty chewing, and trauma to soft tissue due to an impinging bite are all good reasons for considering an orthognathic procedure to resolve these problems. I often see patients who are not happy with the outcome they had with their previous orthodontic treatment when they tried to camouflage their underlying skeletal problem.

I caution patients not to undergo a surgical procedure if they are having any resorption or changes with their condyles, endocrines, or hormones or excessive mandibular growth. Best to wait for the changes to stop occurring and for a period of stability of at least a year prior to considering surgery.

There are several steps involved when one decides to pursue a surgical plan of treatment. Following a detailed consultation with the orthodontist to review all treatment options and it is mutually decided that a surgical procedure would best address the items on the problem list, an appointment is scheduled to have orthodontic treatment initiated. This might consist of clear aligners or orthodontic appliances that are affixed to the teeth. Either way, the teeth must be ideally aligned prior to the surgical procedure.

The alignment phase usually lasts from six months to one year, depending on the severity of the existing malocclusion. The patient is generally referred to the oral surgeon during this initial presurgical alignment phase. The oral surgeon is responsible for contacting the patient's insurance company and getting their medical insurance provider to approve their procedure for coverage. The oral surgeon will also work with the patient to arrange a time for the procedure that is convenient with their schedule. The surgical procedure will take place in an operating room at a hospital with a trained team, including an anesthesiologist, OR staff, and, of course, the oral surgeon.

Generally, after an overnight stay in the ICU, the patient is dismissed to go home. Patients should expect to be off work for two weeks following a procedure. They are on a liquid diet during this time as well. Typically, orthodontic appliances can be removed within three to six months after surgery. Once the orthodontics is completed, the patient then wears some form of retainer, which is either bonded or removable. If any restorative treatment is required, such as crowns or implants, it is best to wait six months to allow for any bite settling or possible surgical relapse to occur. If all that needs to be done is bonding to correct for tooth-size discrepancies, then it can be done much sooner.

Of course, there are possible complications associated with any surgical procedure. The most common with a lower jaw advancement is injury to the inferior alveolar nerve. Damage to the roots of teeth and condylar resorption are also possible. Again, with careful planning and working with an experienced team, complications can be minimized, and the result can be a rewarding experience for the patient. Expectations need to be realistic, with the understanding that not everything may end up perfect.

BEFORE AFTER

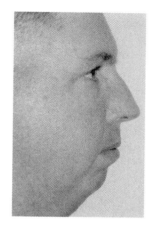 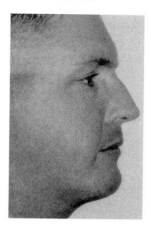

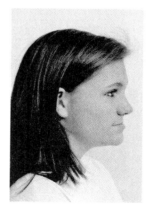 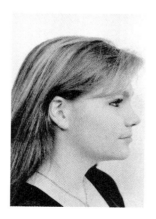

BEFORE AFTER

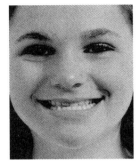
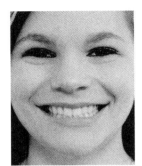

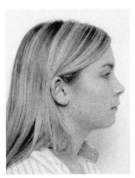
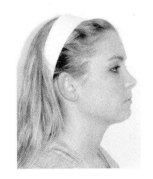

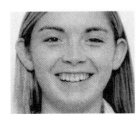
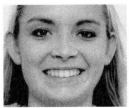

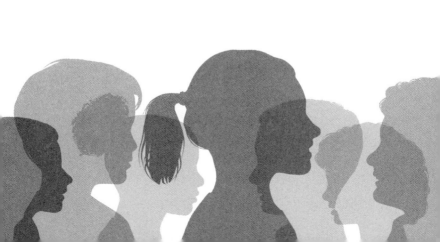

CONCLUSION

I graduated from the UCLA School of Dentistry in 1971 and immediately was accepted to the

University of California at San Francisco, Orthodontic program. The program faculty at that time

was a Who's Who in orthodontics. One of the instructors was Dr. Ronald H Roth! Not only was

he talented, but his purpose and passion in Orthodontics was evident in both his words and actions. When the clinic stopped seeing patients at 5:00 p.m., he would always have a group of us young residents around him, many times until 7:00 p.m. discussing his approach to orthodontics! His passion and compassion were infectious and inspiring.

During my first fifteen years of private practice, I developed a very thriving private practice in orthodontics. I achieved all the outward goals for success. I was a diplomate of the American Board of Orthodontics (at that time fewer than 20 percent of the orthodontists were), associate clinical professor at UCSF, past president of the Alameda County Dental Society, moving "up the chairs" in organized orthodontics, and one of the youngest members of the prestigious Edward H. Angle Society (Dr. Angle is proclaimed by our profession as the Father of Orthodontics). In addition, I had already published many case reports articles in several orthodontic journals. Yes, we all have been there with these material acknowledgments, but we all know there is more to any profession! And it is to be self-critical.

With all these honors and recognitions, I felt I could do more for my patients and improve the efficiency of my care. I sensed that I had a few too many cases that took too long to complete to my high standards, and I was making a few too many "mid-treatment" decisions to complete my cases to these standards. I sensed I did not have clear measurable goals as outlined by Dr. Knight in this book.

In 1990, I decided to "retool" my skills and re united with Dr. Ronald Roth and Dr. Robert Williams, his teaching partner, and devoted the next two years to reexamining diagnosis and treatment planning. The two-year program consisted of seven one-week sessions re-tooling the elements of a complete diagnosis. At that time the course content was much of what Dr. Doug Knight is sharing in this book. We took each of the goals of caring for a patient—functional occlusion, smile esthetics, facial esthetics, periodontal health, and jaw-joint health—and learned measurable treatment goal criteria for each of these goals. Most of these techniques are not taught in orthodontic programs, and if they are, they are presented only in theory during seminars. Many orthodontic residents get "exposed" to these techniques with a sporadic and isolated one-to-three-hour seminar, but residents do not have the opportunity nor time to master these clinical techniques. Mastering these techniques is key to implementing to your patients with success and confidence.

Reconnecting with this post-doctoral course in Functional and Cosmetic Excellence (FACE) and specifically Dr. Roth, forever changed my professional career. Within one year of implementing these tools in my office, my staff and I both noticed a change in the patient treatment outcomes. More patients appeared to finish "on time" with fewer mid-stream decision changes, and more predictable and better outcomes were achieved.

If you're a prospective individual seeking orthodontic treatment for yourself and/or a family member, this book is a must read! It is a most comprehensive overview of what is required to provide the highest quality of orthodontic care available.

You will learn that a FACE-trained and practicing FACE orthodontist recognizes and plans your treatment BEFORE one appliance is placed in the mouth! They look at all the parameters mentioned in this book. Simply stated, this approach is a comprehensive review before any treatment is performed.

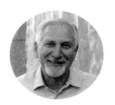

Straty Righellis DDS

Associate Clinical Professor, University
of California at San Francisco

Diplomate, American Board of
Orthodontist

Private Practice, Oakland, California

The FACE philosophy serves as the cornerstone for successful orthodontic treatment. By understanding and applying the principles of occlusion, facial esthetics, and airway anatomy, orthodontists can achieve optimal results, ensuring stable and harmonious dental occlusion for their patients. This book has provided a comprehensive overview of the key components of occlusion, including the relationship between the teeth, muscles, and temporomandibular joints. With this knowledge, orthodontists can diagnose and treat occlusal discrepancies effectively, improving not only the function of the masticatory system but also the esthetics and long-term stability of the dentition.

Furthermore, this book has emphasized the critical connection of how the teeth, lips, and surrounding soft tissues play a vital role in achieving an aesthetically pleasing smile. By considering the FACE principles and their impact on facial balance, orthodontists can create beautiful smiles that enhance the overall facial esthetics and boost their patients' self-confidence.

Another important aspect discussed in this book is the relationship between airway anatomy and obstructions. An obstructed airway can lead to various health issues, including sleep apnea, breathing difficulties, and even cardiovascular problems. By addressing occlusal and skeletal discrepancies, orthodontists can positively influence the upper airway, facilitating proper breathing and improving overall sleep quality. The insights shared in this book will enable orthodontists to approach treatment from a holistic perspective, considering the airway as an integral part of occlusal and orthodontic management.

Lastly, this book has highlighted the significance of interceptive orthodontic treatment in achieving optimal occlusion, facial esthetics, and airway enhancement. Early intervention allows orthodontists to identify and address orthodontic problems at their nascent stages, preventing more severe issues from developing. Through the timely guidance and intervention provided by orthodontists, children can experience improved occlusion, enhanced facial development, and a reduced likelihood of future dental and airway problems. The knowledge and techniques presented in this book will help the reader make better informed decisions for providing the best care for themselves and their children.

In conclusion, the FACE philosophy serves as the foundation for successful orthodontic treatment, promoting optimal dental health, facial esthetics, and airway function, thus establishing the highest standard of care for the overall well-being of the patient it serves.